$10.00

My Pocket Trainer

By Andrew Heckmaster

First Edition, First Printing

ISBN 978-1-304-04033-6

Copyright 2013

Contents

Introduction

After writing _My Training Log_, I realized there was a bit of a hole in what a workout should be. I failed to explain what a good workout was and presumed everyone knew. My deepest apologies for that, but now I have something you can use to fill up your training log. In this book, you will see different types of workout strategies that can be utilized by many people other than martial artists and bodybuilders.

Before performing any type of training regimen, you should consult a doctor to make sure you are healthy enough for physical activity.

Okay, the disclaimer is over and we can talk about the gritty part of exercising. In the following pages, I will explain many body weight exercises, simple bar and dumbbell exercises, and some basic martial arts that anyone can use. I hope you carry this book with you everywhere. It can be very beneficial.

Chapter 1
Pushups

Everyone knows what a pushup is and how to perform it, right? That isn't exactly true. There are many different types of pushups, and they all have specific benefits. First, let's break down what a pushup is.

A standard pushup is a common bodyweight training exercise that builds the pectorals and the triceps. With the variations of pushups in this chapter, you will also be able to build the deltoid and trapezius muscles.

Here is the list of the types of pushups I personally recommend:

Beginner

Incline Pushup

Decline Pushup

Standard Pushup

Incline Military

Decline Military

Standard Military

Incline Wide Fly

Decline Wide Fly

Standard Wide Fly

Incline Diamond

Decline Diamond

Standard Diamond

Advanced

All beginner types from knuckles

Plyometric (Jump) Pushups

Wall Pushups

Single Arm Pushups

The beginner pushups are easily performed by anyone in reasonable shape. The advanced pushups are for those who have conquered the beginner pushups. Once you cease to be challenged by the first list, then move on to the second.

You may be asking yourself why. "Why would I do all of these different types of pushups when I could just do the regular ones?"

The answer is simple. All of them work different muscles. They all work the same groups of muscles, but different individual muscles.

Example: Earlier I mentioned how pushups work the pectorals

(Chest Muscles). A standard pushup will work the middle pectorals while the incline works the lower and the decline works the upper. To get a completely built chest, you have to work from all three heights.

Other types of pushups, like the diamond pushup, will work different muscles. The diamond pushup forces you to work secondary muscles that would not normally be stressed during the standard pushup.

All of them combined will give a complete upper-body workout.

Now, let's go over how to perform some of these:

Incline- Arms elevated on some type of platform like a chair or a couch.

Decline- Legs elevated on some type of platform like a chair or a couch.

Diamond- Buttocks slightly elevated with first fingers and thumbs together in a diamond shape.

Wide Fly- Hands spread apart just past the standard width.

Military- Hands below shoulders.

Plyometric (Jump) - Hands and feet leave the ground.

Wall- The back against the wall with feet in the air.

All of these, with the exception of the diamond and wall pushups, should be performed with the head up and back straight.

No matter what your fitness goal is, use pushups to get you there.

Chapter 2
Abs

Some spend years trying to get defined abdominal muscles. Without a strict diet, this is nearly impossible. Follow a healthy diet plan, and the exercises in this chapter will get you where you want to go.

All of the following exercises will work your upper, middle, and/or lower abdominal muscles.

Flutter Kicks (Legs moving up and down, quickly)

Bicycles

Crunches

Reverse Crunches (Knee to Shoulder)

Cross Crunches (Knee to Elbow)

Sit Ups

Planks (Forearms on the floor)

Hip Thrusts (Hands under butt with feet in the air)

Flutter kicks and Bicycles will wear your legs out. I do not recommend doing these on the same day as any leg activity.

Chapter 3

Legs

There is a seemingly endless amount of leg exercises than can be done by just using your body weight, but there are some that shine brighter than the rest when it comes to effectiveness. In this chapter, you will find the simplest ones that can be performed by almost anyone.

Jogging will be your number one leg workout. It builds cardiovascular strength and calf muscles when done properly.

Remember, when you are jogging, aim to land on the ball or middle of the foot. If you run while striking with the heel, your knees will deteriorate faster.

The rest of the list is simple:

Jumping Jacks

Squats

Lunges

High Knee Raises

Calf Raises

These are all essential to build strength in the legs. Not to mention they can all be done in your living room while you watch television.

All of them can be done fast, and can be aimed at cardiovascular improvement or leg strength.

Chapter 4
The Bar

The bar is a very simple workout tool. You can find one on any park playground, warehouse basement, or for $20 at the local fitness store. A bar is used for two basic things, right? Pull ups and Chin ups are the basics. Like the pushups, these are exercises that can be done in a variety of ways.

Both exercises can be done with a close grip, standard grip, wide grip, or single handed. Be sure to use a chair or stool for assistance with these if you are just starting out.

This marks the end of the cheap and easy training. In the next chapter we will go over some more advanced workouts that require a little more cash, but can be even more rewarding. If you are short on cash, you can skip to chapter 6 to learn how to structure your workouts properly.

Chapter 5

Heavy Bag and Weights

In this chapter, I have put together some things you can use if you can afford a little extra on your equipment. Things you will need to utilize this chapter:

A Heavy Bag with Stand

A Set of Adjustable Dumbbells

A Heavy bag can cost the moon, but you can pick one up with a stand for about $200. For the adjustable dumbbells, I would recommend going with the cheapest set you can find. I got lucky and picked up a set of 5-55lb. adjustable dumbbells for about $60, but others can cost up to $500.

There are a few exercises that I like to use my dumbbells for:

Concentration Curls

Dumbbell Bench Press

Front Raises

Side Raises

Seated Shoulder Press

Preacher Curls

Single Arm Rows

You can easily find examples and photos of how to perform these exercises online or in major bodybuilding publications.

I prefer to use the dumbbells sparingly. It is my opinion that dumbbells can make you slower and less agile if used improperly. If you want to be fast, use less weight and more repetitions. If you want more strength, use more weight and bring down the repetitions.

The heavy bag exercises will be different from almost any other workout. These are more about proper technique and fighting. You can go up and pound on a heavy bag for a while, but you won't improve that much.

To get the most out of a heavy bag routine, follow some of these simple drills to keep sharp and improve your level of fighting and fitness.

#1- *Jab, Cross*

#2- *Hook, Ridge-hand*

#3- *First drill + Front kick*

#4- *Second drill + Roundhouse kick*

These drills stem from my martial arts experience, but they will work for most people.

If you own a heavy bag, be smart about it. Start training with a pair of heavyweight boxing gloves with hand wraps underneath. After you are more experienced, you can move on to just the hand wraps. When you can repeatedly strike the bag with just the wraps, you can slowly progress to just using bare knuckles. This will toughen the knuckles and give you an idea of what a real punch is.

Now, let me break down some of the not-so-obvious techniques you can use on the heavy bag. The first one is the ridge-hand. It is performed in a swinging motion, bringing the hand from the hip like a whip. You will be striking with the inside part of the hand with the thumb tucked underneath the palm.

The second is the front kick. DO NOT kick the bag with the top of the foot. A good heavy bag will break the small bones in your foot if that happens. Instead, stretch the foot out and kick with the ball of the foot. Be sure to point your toes back toward you or they will get broken.

The last of the techniques I want to explain is the roundhouse kick. Hip rotation is the key. Whether it is coming from the back or the front leg, your hips should swing to the bag, not away. It is natural for your arms to work against the leg for balance. Practice by holding on to your shirt to keep this from happening. This is the way you achieve the most power in your kick.

For more information on structuring a workout, please read the next chapter.

Chapter 6

Structuring Workouts

There are three basic ways to workout. Some people are looking to gain speed, some want to gain strength, and others are looking for pure size. All of them have benefits, and I will try my best to help you improve the way you want.

First is speed. Nothing makes you faster than bodyweight exercises. These should be the cornerstone to any training program, and should never be substituted. As I discussed in the first three chapters, there are many forms of bodyweight exercises that you can perform. If I were to put together a training regimen based solely on these, I would split it up like this:

Monday- Pushups

Tuesday-Abs

Wednesday- Legs

Thursday- Pushups

Friday- Abs

Saturday- Legs

These can challenge anyone as long as you perform them fast, efficiently, and with very few breaks in between. If you want to add the bar to this program, you can work it in to your Monday and Thursday workouts.

If you want to add the heavy bag and weights to your training, I suggest putting it together like this:

Monday- Heavy Bag & Upper Body

Tuesday- Heavy Bag & Lower Body

Wednesday- Abs

Thursday- Heavy Bag & Upper Body

Friday- Heavy Bag & Lower Body

Saturday- Abs

If you want to gain strength, five sets of five reps with dumbbells will get you there. For mass, four sets of six to seven reps should work for you. If you want speed, perform three sets of twelve to fifteen reps in RAPID succession. Hopefully you can get where you want to go with that.

There are many other ways to exercise, and you need to choose what is right for you. Don't forget to consult a doctor before beginning any kind of training program. Take care of your body, and it will take care of you.

There is a quote that you should keep in mind before you start thinking your training is too difficult or too strenuous…

"Should you desire the great tranquility, prepare to sweat."

–Hakuin Ekaku

Chapter 7
Nutrition

I am no expert on nutrition, but I will tell you the type of diet that I prefer to use. I realize not everyone can eat organic and healthy all the time. It's a given. Not many of us have that kind of money. So I break it down to the simplest thing.

Protein, Carbs, & Fat

I like to consume one gram of protein per pound of bodyweight at a minimum. For carbs, I prefer to eat potatoes and fruit. I dislike bread, because I feel like I weigh more when I eat it. It slows down my performance when I fight.

I love my vegetables, and I highly recommend eating them all the time. They are a great source of vitamins and minerals and they don't slow me down.

On tournament days, I eat next to nothing and stick to protein in the morning and a piece of fruit every once in a while. This keeps me energized and ready for fighting.

As far as eating fat, I like it. Eggs and bacon in the morning is what I look forward to when I go to bed. You should do some research on the difference between healthy fats and non-healthy fats. You may be surprised.

Also, if you don't have any allergies to nuts, eat them. I eat a lot of them on rest days. I feel they are very important.

Thanks for reading!

Notes:

Notes:

Notes:

Notes:

Notes:

Notes:

www.ingramcontent.com/pod-product-compliance
Lightning Source LLC
Chambersburg PA
CBHW060343290526
45791CB00004B/1507

* 9 7 8 1 3 0 4 0 4 0 3 3 6 *